Infrastructure
Book 2

Also from EATMS Productions

Books on power, survival, women's autonomy, and the systems shaping modern America.

Nonfiction

Analysis of Authoritarian Project 2025

Project 2025: The Blueprint
Project 2025: The List
Project 2025, Christian Dumb Dumbs, & The Republican Agenda
Fascism, Project 2025, & The Pinkprint

Autonomy

Bitcoin for Women
Nostr for Women
Digital Self Defense for Women

Billionaires, Capitalism, and Power

Evil and the Mountain Ungreed
Self Help for American Billionaires
Selfish Steve and the Ivory Tower
Tariffs, Taxes, & Face-Eating Leopards
Ban Billionaires: Fascism Fix

The Epstein Class

The Procurement System
The Shield System
The Respectability System
The Narrative System
The Condition

Fascism, Religion, and Cultural Control

Self Help for the Manosphere
Fascism 2025: and the winner is
Fascism & the Perverts & the Greed Virus
Christian Fascism Marriage Book
Tyranny, Table Manners, & Tiramisu

Guides for Women's Autonomy and Protection

How to Survive in Post-America as a Woman
Project 2025 American Drag: Women's Study Bible FTP
4B – Burn, Ban, Boycott, Build (4B Movement)
4B OG – So No Go GYN (4B Movement)
I'm Glad He's Dead

Modern Rewrites for Women

Stoic Principles Reimagined
Siddhartha Reimagined
The Prince Reimagined for Women
The Art of War Reimagined for Women
The Jungle Reimagined
The Constitution Reimagined for Women

Response to Heritage Foundation's New Project 2025:

Saving America by Saving the Family: A Foundation for the Next 250 Years
The Blueprint II
The List II
The Pinkprint II
The Grayprint Inferno

Fiction

Dystopian Stories of Resistance and Collapse

Propaganda Paige & the Missing Prosperity
Propaganda Paige & the TIDE Manifesto
Propaganda Paige & the Shadow Cartographers
Propaganda Paige & the Prosperity Alliance
Propaganda Paige & the Shattered Truth
Propaganda Paige & the Rising TIDE
Propaganda Paige & the Last Bastion
Propaganda Paige & the Dawn of Prosperity
Project 2025: Dorian — The Last Men
Project 2025: Boy — A Last Men Novel

Survival Guides
For Women in Authoritarian America

Civics
How American Government Actually Works
Parties, Ideologies, & Promises vs Outcomes
Elections, Voting, & Leverage
Power, Money, Media, & the Courts

Infrastructure
Power & Heat
Water & Waste
Food & Supply
Shelter & Movement

Machine Learning
AI, Bitcoin, Nostr for Women
AI, Safety, & Security for Women
AI, Anxiety, & Health for Women
AI, Kids, & Family Safety for Women
AI, Creativity, & Personal Expression for Women
AI, Independent Work, & Parallel Power for Women

Religious Authority as a Governing System
Authority Without Consent
Law as Revelation
The Family as Enforcement Unit
Education, Indoctrination, & Withdrawal
Economics of Submission
Theocratic Convergence

Social Systems
Emotional Labor for Women
Household Power for Women
Workplace Power for Women
Medical Bias for Women
Aging Systems for Women
Recovery Systems for Women

Water & Waste

A Survival Guide for Women in Authoritarian America

by
Alice Horton
& Helena Hemmings

intro by
Esme Mees

EATMS
PRODUCTIONS

This title is part of an ongoing body of work. All EATMS Productions titles, across all series, authors, and formats, are components of a single connected project.

This book is a work of opinion and creative interpretation. While some names and events may be referenced or alluded to, any claims made are based on publicly available information and are intended as satire, parody, or commentary on societal and political issues. The content should not be interpreted as factual assertions about any individual or entity. The author does not intend to defraud, defame, or mislead, and encourages readers to form their own conclusions. Any resemblance to real persons, living or dead, is purely coincidental unless explicitly noted otherwise.

ISBN: 978-1-966014-64-5

Cover, interior design by: Esme Mees

eatms@pm.me
www.eatms.me

Check out EATMS Underground:
https://tinyurl.com/eatmsNOSTR

Printed in the United States of America.

Pure air. Pure water. Efficient drainage. Cleanliness. Light.
Without these, no house can be healthy.

— Florence Nightingale

Table of Contents

How to Use This Guide

This is a book about water and waste, which means it is a book about two things every household depends on without wanting to think about them. Clean water comes in. Used water and waste go out. When both work, they are invisible. When either fails, the house changes fast. This book is part of the EATMS Infrastructure Series, a survival guide for women in authoritarian America, where these systems are aging and left for households to handle alone.

You can read this book straight through, or go directly to the chapter matching what is happening now. If the tap water looks, smells, or tastes wrong, start with water quality. If a boil water notice arrives, start with boil notices and emergency water. If a toilet will not flush or there is a sewage smell, start with sewage or septic systems. If the basement is wet, start with flooding, drainage, and mold. If the water bill jumped or a shutoff notice arrived, start with leaks, bills, and shutoffs. If a landlord is delaying a water repair, start with repair responsibility and documentation.

Each chapter begins with ordinary material life: a tap, a toilet, a drain, a basement, a bill. Then it moves outward to explain what is happening underneath, where the subtitle stops being abstract. Where does the water come from. Where does waste go. Who owns the pipes. Who is responsible for repair. Who decides whether a problem is urgent or someone else's burden, once oversight has weakened. From there, each chapter returns to what you can check, document, ask, prepare, or refuse to carry alone.

This is not a plumbing manual. It will not teach you to replace a pipe, rebuild a toilet, or design a treatment plant. It is not a prepper manual built around the fantasy that every household can become water-independent. Most people cannot, and should not have to. This book assumes you live inside systems you did not build and cannot fix yourself.

At the end of every chapter, you will find a short action list in four parts. What to Notice covers early signs that something may be wrong. What to Check covers concrete things you can look at, test, ask about, or write down. What to Do Before Crisis covers realistic preparation, such as knowing where the shutoff valve is or documenting a problem before it becomes an emergency.

The fourth part is What Not to Waste Energy On. Water and waste problems carry shame, panic, disgust, and blame. People respond by buying things they do not need, hiding problems too long, or quietly trying to solve failures that belong to landlords, utilities, or policy. That section helps separate what is yours from what was always a public failure handed to you.

The final chapter brings the book together into the EATMS Water and Waste Plan. The goal is not control you do not have. It is a clearer map, fewer surprises, better questions, and a steadier way to move through water, plumbing, sewage, or sanitation failure without starting from zero.

Introduction

There is a moment most people never think about until it stops happening. You turn on the tap, and water comes out. You flush the toilet, and the water and everything in it disappears, quietly, somewhere else. You wash your hands, fill a glass, run laundry, rinse dishes, clean a child, help an elder bathe, or make food without thinking of any of it as infrastructure. It just is, until one day it is not. This book is part of the EATMS Infrastructure Series, a survival guide for women in authoritarian America, where public oversight keeps loosening even as the systems beneath it get privatized, underfunded, and left to fail quietly.

Women tend to meet this system earlier than most infrastructure stories admit, and they meet it from the inside. A water problem rarely announces itself as a water problem first. It shows up as laundry that cannot get done, a sink full of dishes, a baby bottle that needs washing, a bathroom that cannot be used, a smell that will not go away, or a basement that stays damp longer than it should. The people managing those problems day to day are very often women, and they are managing them long before anyone calls it a public failure rather than a private one.

This book is about two things that have to work together. Clean water has to come into your home, and used water and waste have to leave it safely. Most people think first about the water coming out of the tap, but the other side matters just as much. A toilet that will not flush, a septic system that backs up, a sewer line that fails, or a basement that floods with water and sewage mixed together can make a home unsafe just as quickly as contaminated drinking water can.

Both halves of this system are easy to ignore until they fail, and both are shaped by decisions made far from your kitchen. Safe water depends on pipes, testing, treatment, funding, and what happens when contamination is found. Safe waste removal depends on sewers, septic systems, drainage, maintenance, landlords, utilities, and public agencies with authority that keeps getting trimmed back as the systems it oversees keep aging. None of that is visible from the sink. All of it can end up there anyway.

Water and sanitation are not just home maintenance topics. They are public health, and public health depends on systems being maintained, funded, and held accountable, exactly the kind of commitment that erodes first under the conditions this book describes. When maintenance is deferred, utilities are privatized, regulations go unenforced, landlords ignore repairs, and local governments are underfunded, the risk does not disappear. It moves into corroding pipes, untested wells, overloaded sewers, flooded basements, moldy walls, shutoff notices, and homes where someone still has to cook, clean, bathe, caregive, and keep people from getting sick.

That someone is not evenly distributed. A boil water notice means something different to a household with an infant, an elder, immune compromise, or no money for bottled water. A sewer backup is one kind of crisis for a homeowner with insurance and a restoration company. For a renter, it can mean days of fighting a landlord just to get the danger acknowledged and documented.

This book is written for municipal water and private wells, sewer systems and septic systems, renters and homeowners, rural households and city households, fragile budgets and caregiving-heavy homes, living where clean water in and safe waste out is no longer something to take for granted. The details differ, but the core questions are the same. Where does your water come from? Where does your waste go? Who is responsible when something fails? What can you check, report, and document? What is simply not yours to fix?

The chapters ahead cover water access and quality, private wells and municipal systems, boil notices, shutoffs, unaffordable bills, leaks, toilets, drains, sewer and septic systems, flooding, stormwater, mold, caregiving risk, documentation, and household planning. They look at water and waste as lived household events, not just technical problems.

None of this will give you total control over the systems your home depends on. No book can do that, and any book that promises it is selling you something. What this book offers is a clearer map of how those systems work, better questions to ask when something goes wrong, fewer false assumptions about your responsibility, less shame about problems never yours to begin with, and a steadier way through water and waste failures.

— Esme Mees, Summer 2026

~1
Water Is Survival

You turn on the tap to fill a pot, and the water comes out clean, the right temperature, exactly as expected. You flush the toilet and everything in it disappears, carried somewhere out of sight, out of mind. Someone runs a load of towels after a stomach bug moves through the house. Someone fills a glass of water at midnight without turning on a light. None of this registers as a system working. It just happens, the same way the floor holds your weight, until the day it doesn't.

Then the water comes out brown, or smells like rotten eggs, or barely trickles from the faucet no matter how far you turn the handle. Or the toilet doesn't flush right, and a few hours later the bathtub starts gurgling every time someone runs the washing machine. Or a notice goes up telling everyone in the area not to drink the tap water until further testing is done. In that moment, the thing that felt like nothing becomes the only thing anyone in the house can think about.

Water in a home is not just drinking water, even though that is usually the first thing people picture. It is the water used to cook dinner, to wash hands before handling food, to bathe a child or an elderly parent, to run a dishwasher, to do laundry, to mix infant formula, to flush a toilet, to clean a wound, to rinse the cup someone uses for their medication. Take water away, or make it unsafe, and all of those small daily tasks stop being routine and start being decisions, often urgent ones, made by whoever in the household is paying attention.

The other half of this system gets even less attention, and that is everything involved in getting waste safely out of the house. Drains, toilets, sewer lines, septic tanks, sump pumps: all of it exists for one purpose, which is to make sure that what the household produces does not stay inside the household. When that system works, nobody thinks about it. When it fails, a clogged drain or a backed-up sewer line can turn a bathroom or a basement into a place that is not just unpleasant but unsafe, especially once mold or standing wastewater is involved.

So there are two sides to this, and both can fail independently. Clean water has to come in. Waste has to go out. A household can be put at risk by no water at all, by water that looks fine but isn't, by water that is simply too expensive to keep running, by a pipe that freezes and bursts, by a drain that backs up, by a septic system that fails, or by a basement that floods and stays wet long enough for mold to take hold. None of these are rare or exotic problems. They are the kind of thing that happens in ordinary homes, on ordinary streets, more often than most people realize until it happens to them.

When something on either side goes wrong, the work of dealing with it tends to land in a predictable place. Someone notices the smell from the basement before anyone else does. Someone decides whether the tap water is safe enough to use for the baby's bottle today, or whether it's worth the trip to buy bottled water instead. Someone strips the bed and starts a second load of laundry after an elderly parent has an accident, and then has to think about where that water goes and whether the bathroom is safe to use while things dry out. This work is not assigned because of biology, and it is not a sign of anyone's personal failing. It falls to whoever is already doing the daily logistics of the household, and in most households, that is a woman, whether she is doing it with a partner or entirely on her own.

None of this starts with the household, even though the household feels it first. It starts with old pipes, water mains that should have been replaced years ago, utilities that answer to shareholders instead of residents, landlords who ignore slow drains or failing water heaters, and groundwater contaminated by something upstream. The household ends up living with all of these decisions, but it made none of them.

This book is not going to turn you into a plumber, and it is not going to suggest that you should handle a sewer backup or contaminated well on your own with the right tools and enough determination. What it will do is help you understand what your home depends on, what you can reasonably check, what is worth documenting, who to call when something goes wrong, and which parts of the problem were never yours to solve.

The same water or waste problem does not land the same way in every household. A boil water notice is a minor inconvenience for someone with a car, savings, and an otherwise healthy household. It is a much bigger problem for someone with an infant, immune compromise, wound care needs, or a private well with no clear answer about whether the water was affected. A sewer backup is one kind of crisis for a homeowner with insurance and a restoration company. For a renter, it can mean days or weeks of trying to get a landlord to acknowledge that sewage came up through the floor, let alone clean it properly and deal with the mold that follows.

The first step through any of this is not panic, and it is not buying things. It is making the invisible visible. Where does your water actually come from, and is it municipal water or a private well that someone is responsible for testing? Where does your waste actually go when it leaves the house, into a city sewer system or a septic system in the yard? Do you know where the main water shutoff is, and have you ever had to find it in the dark? Are there any drains, toilets, or corners of a basement that have already been quietly trying to get your attention? And if the water stopped tomorrow, or became unsafe, or the waste stopped leaving, who in your household would feel that first, and how fast? Those questions are where the rest of this book begins.

Chapter 1 Action List: Water Is Survival

What to Notice

- Any change in your water's smell, color, taste, or pressure, even a small one
- Drains that are slow to empty, gurgle, or have started to smell
- A toilet that clogs repeatedly or flushes weaker than it used to
- Damp spots, staining, standing water, or a musty smell anywhere in the home
- Whether anyone in the household depends on clean water for medication, formula, or medical care
- Whether your water bill has been creeping up without an obvious reason
- Whether a landlord has been told about a water or drainage problem and how they responded

What to Check

- Whether your home is on municipal water or a private well, and who is responsible for testing it
- Whether your waste goes to a city sewer system or a septic system on the property
- Where the main water shutoff valve is located, and whether you can actually reach it
- Your most recent water bills, looking for sudden increases that might point to a hidden leak
- Your lease, if you rent, for language about who is responsible for plumbing repairs

- Whether your local water utility has a website or hotline for outages, boil notices, or billing questions
- Whether anyone nearby on a private well has had it tested recently, if you're on one too

What to Do Before Crisis

- Write down your water provider's name, account number, and a phone number for emergencies or outages
- Locate your main shutoff valve and make sure at least one other adult in the household knows where it is
- Keep a small, realistic amount of drinking water on hand, enough for a day or two if possible
- Start a simple written record of any leaks, odors, stains, or drainage issues, with dates and photos
- If you're on a private well, find out when it was last tested and what it was tested for
- Save your local health department and public works contact information somewhere accessible without power

What Not to Waste Energy On

- Blaming yourself for not understanding how the plumbing in your home works
- Buying expensive water filters or treatment systems before you know what the actual problem is
- Treating a landlord's delay or neglect as evidence that you failed to manage your household

- Assuming a sewer or septic problem is embarrassing or something to hide rather than report
- Comparing your situation to households with more savings, more space, or more control over their housing
- Trying to fix a municipal or systemic problem privately, on your own, before asking who is actually responsible

~2
Drinking Water

You fill a glass at the kitchen sink, the way you have a thousand times before, and you take a sip without thinking about it. Then you stop. Something is off. Maybe it tastes faintly like a swimming pool, or like metal, or like nothing at all in a way that feels wrong. Maybe it's perfectly clear, perfectly normal looking, and you drink it anyway because it looks fine, and looking fine is the only test most of us ever apply.

That's the first thing worth understanding about drinking water. The way it looks tells you almost nothing. Water can be completely clear, cold, and pleasant to drink, and still contain things that matter for your health. And water can look or smell a little off and still be perfectly safe. Sight, taste, and smell are not reliable tests, and most households have no other way to check, which means most people are trusting a system they've never seen and don't fully understand.

For most people in this country, that system is municipal water. In plain terms, this means your water comes from a source, usually a river, lake, reservoir, or a set of wells the utility controls, and it gets pulled into a treatment plant. At the plant, it goes through a series of steps designed to remove particles, kill bacteria and viruses, and adjust the chemistry so the water won't corrode the pipes it travels through afterward. From there it goes into a network of underground pipes, sometimes decades old, sometimes over a century old, that carries it to your home. By the time it reaches your tap, it has been treated, but it has also traveled through a lot of infrastructure that the treatment plant has no control over.

The other major source is a private well. If your water comes from a well, there is no treatment plant, no utility testing it on a schedule, and usually no one checking it at all unless you arrange for that yourself. A well pulls water directly from the ground, from an aquifer that may be shallow or deep, clean or affected by whatever sits near it: a septic system, a farm field, an old gas station, a landfill from decades ago that nobody remembers anymore. Well water can be excellent. It can also be quietly carrying something that has been there for years, completely undetectable without a test.

Both of these systems can fail in ways that don't show up as a dramatic event. A water main break is obvious. But the slow leaching of lead from old pipes, the gradual buildup of certain chemicals in a well, the corrosion happening inside your own home's plumbing: none of that comes with a smell or a warning. It just accumulates, quietly, in the water you've been drinking and cooking with the entire time.

This is where testing comes in, and it's worth being honest about what testing can and can't tell you. A water test can tell you whether specific things are present, at the time the sample was taken, in the amounts that test was designed to detect. It cannot tell you that your water is generally safe forever, and it cannot test for everything, because there is no single test that covers every possible contaminant. If you're on municipal water, your utility is required to test for a defined list of substances and to publish the results, usually once a year, in something called a water quality report or consumer confidence report. If you're on a well, none of that happens unless you pay for it yourself, and most people never do, often because they don't know they should, or because a basic test costs money they don't have to spend on something that isn't an obvious emergency.

Bottled water gets brought up a lot in conversations about water safety, and it's worth being clear about its limits. Bottled water can be useful in a short-term situation, like a boil water notice or a contamination event, when you need something safe to drink right away. It is not a long-term household water strategy. It's expensive, it's heavy, it requires storage space many households don't have, and it does nothing to address whatever the actual problem with your water might be. If your water is unsafe, bottled water buys you time. It doesn't buy you a solution.

Filtration sits in a similar place. A pitcher filter, a faucet attachment, or a whole-house filtration system can reduce certain contaminants, but only the ones that specific filter is designed to remove. A filter that handles chlorine taste and odor does nothing for lead. A filter rated for lead may do nothing for bacteria. Filters need their cartridges replaced on a schedule, and an old cartridge can sometimes make water worse instead of better. None of this means filters are useless. It means a filter is only as useful as your understanding of what it actually does, and buying one before you know what your water's actual issue is can mean spending money on the wrong problem entirely.

One of the more frustrating parts of all this is how confusing the official information can be. A water quality report from your utility might be sent in the mail, or it might only be available online, in a format full of technical terms and numbers compared against limits that are never explained. A boil water notice might use language that sounds urgent without telling you how long it will last or what it actually covers. For someone managing a household, working, caring for kids or an elder, and already stretched thin, decoding a document like that on top of everything else can feel like one more task nobody has time for.

It's also worth saying plainly that in a lot of communities, trust in the water itself has been damaged, and not without reason. There have been places where officials said the water was safe when it wasn't, where testing was delayed, where residents reported problems for months or years before anyone with authority acknowledged them. If you live somewhere that has been through something like that, or somewhere where people talk about the water with suspicion, that suspicion didn't come from nowhere. It doesn't mean every glass of tap water everywhere is dangerous. It means that for a lot of people, the assumption that "the water is fine because no one said otherwise" has already been tested and found wanting.

That loss of trust changes the work inside a household. It means someone has to decide whether the notice is clear enough, whether the filter is doing anything useful, whether the landlord is being honest, whether the county website has been updated, whether the stain in the sink matters, and whether the child, elder, or sick person in the house needs a different answer than everyone else. That is not paranoia. It is the labor that appears when public confidence has been spent badly and ordinary people are left trying to sort risk from reassurance at the kitchen tap.

None of this is meant to make you afraid of your own kitchen sink. It's meant to replace a vague, background unease with something more specific: knowing where your water actually comes from, knowing what information exists about it and where to find it, and knowing what a strange taste, smell, or color might be worth paying attention to versus what's probably nothing. That's a very different position to be in than simply hoping the water is fine because it always has been.

Chapter 2 Action List: Drinking Water

What to Notice

- Any change in taste, smell, color, or clarity of your tap water, even if it seems minor
- Sediment, cloudiness, or a film that appears in water after it sits in a glass
- A metallic, chemical, or "swimming pool" taste that wasn't there before
- Whether your water pressure has changed recently, especially a sudden drop
- Whether anyone in the household has had unexplained stomach issues that seem tied to drinking water
- Whether you've ever received a water quality report and what you did with it
- Whether your area has a history of water quality complaints or distrust

What to Check

- Whether your home is on municipal water or a private well
- If municipal, find your utility's most recent water quality or consumer confidence report
- If on a well, find out when it was last tested, by whom, and for what
- Whether your home's plumbing includes any older pipes, especially if the home was built before the 1980s
- What kind of filter, if any, your household currently uses and what it's actually rated to remove

- Whether your local health department has any current advisories for your area
- Whether your water utility has a customer service or emergency line saved somewhere

What to Do Before Crisis

- Request or download a copy of your most recent water quality report, even if everything seems fine
- If on a well, look into the cost of a basic water test through your local health department, often cheaper than private labs
- Write down your water utility's name, account number, and emergency contact information
- If you use a filter, check the replacement schedule and write down when the cartridge was last changed
- Keep a small supply of bottled or stored water on hand for short-term use, sized to your household
- Save your local health department's contact information somewhere accessible

What Not to Waste Energy On

- Buying an expensive filtration system before you know what, if anything, is actually in your water
- Assuming clear, good-tasting water means there is nothing to be concerned about
- Assuming a strange taste or smell automatically means something dangerous is happening

- Feeling embarrassed about not understanding water quality reports, which are genuinely hard to read
- Treating a private well's safety as something only "rural people" need to think about
- Trying to solve a contamination concern on your own before contacting your utility or health department

~3
Wells & Cities

In one house, the power goes out during a storm, and along with the lights, the water stops too. Nothing comes out of the tap, not even a trickle, because the well that supplies this house runs on an electric pump, and the pump runs on electricity that is currently not coming. The toilet still has one flush left in the tank, and that's it. A few miles away, in town, the power is out too, but the water is still running, because the city system has its own backup power and gravity doing a lot of the work. That household has water. It also has a notice on the city's website, easy to miss, saying that a water main broke that morning and the water should be boiled until further notice. Neither household has it easy. They just have different problems, and neither of them chose which one they got.

This is the real difference between a private well and a municipal water system, and it's worth understanding clearly, because a lot of people carry assumptions about which one is "safer" that don't hold up once you look closely.

A private well is exactly what it sounds like: a hole drilled into the ground, deep enough to reach water-bearing rock or soil, called an aquifer, with a pump that pulls that water up and pushes it into the house. There's usually a pressure tank nearby that keeps water available between pump cycles, so the pump isn't running every single time someone turns on a faucet. If the household has a water softener or filtration system, that's part of the setup too. All of this sits on the property, and all of it belongs to the household. There is no utility bill for the water itself, no monthly charge for the water flowing through the pipes. But there is also no one else checking any of it. No one tests it on a schedule. No one inspects the pump. No one tells you when the pressure tank is failing until it fails. If something breaks, the cost and the responsibility land entirely on whoever owns that property.

And because the pump runs on electricity, a well household is tied to the power grid in a way that isn't always obvious until the power goes out. No electricity means no pump, which means no water at all: not for drinking, not for the toilet, not for washing hands, not for anything, until the power comes back or there's a generator running. This is one of the most overlooked dependencies in rural households, and it matters most exactly when it's most inconvenient: during storms, outages, and emergencies, when water suddenly becomes one more thing that isn't working.

A municipal water system works completely differently, and on a much larger scale. Somewhere, often miles away, there's a source: a river, a lake, a reservoir, or a collection of wells that belong to the utility rather than to any individual household. That water gets pulled into a treatment plant, where it's filtered, disinfected, and chemically balanced before it's pushed into a network of underground pipes that branch out across the whole service area, eventually reaching your house. Many systems also use elevated water towers or storage tanks, which help maintain pressure and provide a buffer if the treatment plant has to shut down temporarily. This is part of why some municipal systems can keep water flowing for a while even during a power outage. Gravity and stored pressure can keep things moving for a time, even when the pumps that normally help aren't running.

On municipal water, someone else owns the infrastructure, someone else is required to test the water on a regular schedule, and someone else is responsible for fixing a water main when it breaks. That sounds like a clear advantage, and in many ways it is. But it also means your water is part of a system you have zero control over and very little visibility into. The pipes carrying water to your house might be the same pipes that were installed when the neighborhood was built, which in many American cities means pipes that are fifty, eighty, or even over a hundred years old. Some of those pipes are made of materials that are no longer considered safe, including lead. The treatment plant might be doing everything right, and the water might still pick up contaminants on its way to your tap, from the pipes it passes through on the way.

This is the part that surprises people: being on municipal water doesn't mean your water is automatically safer than well water, and being on a well doesn't automatically mean you're at higher risk. Both systems have weak points. A well's weak point is usually testing, maintenance, and power dependency. A municipal system's weak point is often aging infrastructure, funding, and how honestly problems get communicated once they're found.

Geography changes the picture too, in ways that aren't always obvious. In rural areas, if something goes wrong with a well, the household is often on its own, sometimes a long drive from the nearest well contractor, and often facing repair costs that can run into thousands of dollars for something like a failed pump or a well that needs to be drilled deeper. There's no neighbor to borrow water from, and often no backup plan beyond bottled water from a store that might be twenty minutes away.

In cities, especially in older neighborhoods, the problem looks different. The water utility might be a city department, or it might be a private company that bought the water system years ago and now answers primarily to investors. Either way, decisions about which pipes get replaced, and in what order, are made somewhere far from any individual household, often based on budget constraints that have been building for decades. Neighborhoods with less political power, often lower-income and often with larger populations of color, have historically been last in line for infrastructure upgrades, and that pattern doesn't disappear just because someone writes a press release about it.

Renters occupy an especially uncertain position in all of this, regardless of whether the building is on a well or municipal water. If the water tastes strange, or the pressure is low, or there's a notice about the building's water system, a renter usually has no direct relationship with the utility and no authority to fix anything. The landlord is the one who gets the notices, who decides whether to act on them, and who controls whether tenants even find out there's a problem at all. A renter on a well is in an even more layered situation, because the landlord may be the only one who knows when the well was last tested, if it ever was.

Mobile homes and manufactured housing communities add another layer entirely. Many of these communities have their own small water systems, sometimes called community wells or package treatment systems, which are technically regulated but often operate with minimal oversight and minimal funding. Residents may pay a water fee to the park owner without ever knowing whether the system serving their homes is being maintained, tested, or even legally compliant.

The point of laying all this out isn't to make either option, well or municipal, sound hopeless. It's to push back against the idea that your water source alone tells you whether you're safe. "I'm on city water, so it's fine" and "I'm on a well, so at least I know what's in it" are both assumptions that can be wrong, and both can lead to the same outcome: nobody checking anything until something forces the issue. What actually matters is knowing which system you're part of, what its specific weak points are, who is responsible for maintaining it, and what you can realistically find out about its condition before you need that information in a hurry.

Chapter 3 Action List: Wells & Cities

What to Notice

- Whether your water pressure or flow changes during storms, outages, or extreme weather
- Whether your well pump makes unusual sounds, cycles more often than normal, or runs constantly
- Any notices from your municipal utility about main breaks, boil advisories, or service changes
- Whether your water tastes, smells, or looks different after heavy rain or after any nearby construction
- Whether your home is in a mobile home park, manufactured housing community, or small private system
- Whether you've ever seen a water bill, water report, or well record for your home
- Whether neighbors on the same well or same water system have mentioned any problems

What to Check

- Whether your home's water comes from a private well, a municipal system, or a small community system
- If on a well, where the pump, pressure tank, and any treatment equipment are located
- If on a well, whether the household has a backup plan for water during a power outage
- If on municipal water, the age of the neighborhood's water mains and whether lead service lines have been an issue locally

- If renting, whether the landlord has shared any water testing records, notices, or system information
- Whether your area's water utility is publicly owned or privately operated
- Whether your community has a history of water infrastructure complaints, especially in lower-income neighborhoods

What to Do Before Crisis

- If on a well, find out the make, model, and approximate age of your pump and pressure tank
- If on a well, store a realistic amount of drinking water for outages, since no power means no water
- If on municipal water, sign up for any text or email alert system your utility offers for outages and notices
- Write down whether your home has lead service lines, or how to find out, especially in older buildings
- If renting, request in writing any water testing records or notices the landlord has received
- Identify the nearest alternative water source, such as a relative's home or a store, in case yours is unavailable

What Not to Waste Energy On

- Assuming municipal water is automatically safer than well water, or the reverse

- Assuming a well household has "opted out" of public systems and therefore has no risk
- Feeling like you should have already known the age or condition of your home's water infrastructure
- Blaming yourself for living in a mobile home, rental, or older neighborhood with aging infrastructure
- Trying to personally fix or test for problems that are the utility's or landlord's legal responsibility
- Assuming a working tap today means the underlying system is in good condition

~4 Contamination

A letter comes in the mail, or a notice gets posted online, or a neighbor mentions it in passing, and it has a word in it that lands differently than other words. Lead. PFAS. Nitrates. E. coli. Arsenic. The word might be unfamiliar, or it might be one you've heard before in a news story about some other town, some other water system, somewhere that always felt far away. Now it has your address on it, or your well, or your neighborhood, and you don't know what it means for the water you've been drinking, cooking with, and giving to your kids for years.

This chapter is about that moment, and about what comes before and after it. Contamination is one of the most frightening words in the water world, partly because it covers so many different things, and partly because most people have no framework for understanding what any of it actually means for their household. The goal here isn't to turn you into a chemist. It's to give you enough of a map that when one of these words shows up in your life, you have somewhere to put it.

The first thing worth separating out is that contamination is a health issue, not a cleanliness issue. Water that is contaminated doesn't necessarily look dirty, smell bad, or taste off. Some contaminants are completely undetectable without a lab test. This is uncomfortable, because it means the usual signals people rely on, the ones this book has talked about in earlier chapters, don't apply here. A glass of water can look perfectly clear and still contain something that matters for your health, especially over years of exposure.

It helps to think of contamination in a few rough categories, because the source, the risk, and the response are different for each.

The first category is biological: bacteria, viruses, and parasites. This is usually the kind of contamination behind a boil water notice, and it's also the most common issue with private wells, especially wells that are old, poorly sealed, or located too close to a septic system, livestock, or flooding. Biological contamination tends to cause illness relatively quickly, often within a day or two of exposure, with symptoms like stomach upset, diarrhea, or vomiting. It's also the kind of contamination that boiling water actually fixes, which is why boil notices exist.

The second category is what gets called "legacy" contamination, things that got into pipes, soil, or groundwater a long time ago and are still there. Lead is the most well-known example. Lead doesn't come from the water source itself, in most cases. It comes from old pipes, old solder, and old fixtures, especially in homes and water systems built before the late 1980s. Lead doesn't smell or taste like anything, and it doesn't cause sudden illness. Its damage is cumulative, especially in children, where even low levels of exposure over time can affect brain development. This is why lead testing is often recommended for homes with young children or pregnant women, and why the age of a home's plumbing matters even if the water utility's source water is completely clean.

The third category is industrial and chemical contamination, and this is where PFAS usually comes up. PFAS stands for a large group of manufactured chemicals that were used for decades in things like nonstick cookware, firefighting foam, water-resistant fabrics, and food packaging. They don't break down easily, which is part of why they're sometimes called "forever chemicals," and they've ended up in groundwater near military bases, airports, manufacturing sites, and landfills across the country. PFAS contamination is almost always tied to a specific source nearby, even if that source isn't obvious or hasn't been publicly identified yet. Like lead, PFAS doesn't change how water looks, smells, or tastes, and its health effects are about long-term exposure rather than a sudden illness.

The fourth category is agricultural, and the word that comes up most often here is nitrates. Nitrates come from fertilizer and from animal waste, and they can seep into groundwater in farming areas, especially affecting private wells near fields or livestock operations. Nitrates are a particular concern for infants, because high levels can interfere with how a baby's blood carries oxygen, a condition sometimes called blue baby syndrome. This is one of the few contamination risks where the danger is concentrated almost entirely in one group, infants under six months old, while being far less of a concern for older children and adults.

There's also a broader category that's harder to name simply: everything else that can end up in groundwater or surface water because of how land gets used. Old gas stations with leaking underground tanks. Dry cleaners that used solvents decades ago. Industrial sites that closed down without proper cleanup. Pesticides from nearby farms or even from lawns. None of these show up on a standard water test unless someone specifically tests for them, which usually only happens if there's a known reason to look.

What ties all of this together is a pattern that shows up again and again: contamination is rarely something a household creates, and it's almost never something a household can fully verify on its own. The well was already there when the contamination happened. The pipes were installed before the household moved in. The factory closed before anyone living nearby today was born. And yet the household is the one drinking the water, bathing the kids in it, and trying to figure out what, if anything, needs to change.

This is also where a particular kind of dismissal tends to show up, and it's worth naming directly. When people, especially women, raise concerns about water quality, a common response is some version of "it's probably fine" or "we've always used this water and we're fine," offered before anyone has actually tested anything. Sometimes that reassurance comes from a landlord who doesn't want to deal with a plumbing problem. Sometimes it comes from a local official who doesn't want to deal with a public relations problem. Sometimes it comes from a relative who genuinely believes it, because nothing has gone wrong yet that anyone noticed. None of that is the same as an actual answer, and "probably fine" is not a test result.

The people most affected by contamination, in terms of health risk, are often the people least likely to be centered in how these issues get discussed. Pregnant women and infants face risks from lead and nitrates that don't apply the same way to healthy adults. Children absorb more, relative to their body weight, than adults do, and their developing systems are more vulnerable to long-term exposure. Elders and people with existing health conditions may be more affected by contaminants that wouldn't bother a healthy adult much at all. If you're managing a household that includes any of these people, contamination isn't an abstract policy question. It's a question about the specific people in your home.

Testing is the only way to move from "I don't know" to "I know," but it's worth being realistic about what testing involves. A basic test for bacteria is usually inexpensive and often available through a local health department, especially for well owners. Testing for something like lead, PFAS, or a specific pesticide is more expensive and usually requires sending a sample to a specialized lab. You don't need to test for everything at once. What matters is testing for the things that are actually relevant to your situation: your home's age and plumbing if lead is a concern, your well's location if nitrates or bacteria are a concern, or a known nearby contamination source if PFAS has been found in your area.

Filters come up again here, and the same caution from the last chapter applies, with more weight. A filter that isn't certified to remove a specific contaminant does nothing about that contaminant, no matter how expensive or impressive it looks. Some filters can make a real difference for lead or certain chemicals, but only if they're the right kind, installed correctly, and maintained on schedule. A filter bought out of fear, without knowing what's actually in the water, can create a false sense of security that's worse than knowing nothing at all, because it stops people from asking the next question.

If contamination is identified, documentation matters more than it might for an ordinary plumbing problem. Test results, official notices, correspondence with a utility or landlord, and photos of notices posted in a building can all matter later, whether for a renter trying to get a landlord to act, a homeowner seeking assistance, or a community trying to hold a utility or local government accountable. Contamination problems often take years to be acknowledged publicly, and the households that are believed are often the ones that kept records before anyone official was willing to.

None of this is meant to leave you feeling like every glass of water might be hiding something dangerous. Most water, most of the time, in most places, does not contain dangerous levels of any of this. But "most of the time, in most places" is not the same as "your water, right now," and the only way to close that gap is information: your water source, your home's plumbing age, your area's known issues, and what a real test would involve if you ever needed one.

Chapter 4 Action List: Contamination

What to Notice

- Any official notice, letter, or news report mentioning contamination in your water system or area
- Whether your home was built before the late 1980s, which affects the likelihood of lead pipes or solder
- Whether you live near a farm, livestock operation, factory, airport, military base, or old gas station
- Reassurances about water safety that aren't backed by an actual test result
- Whether anyone in your household is pregnant, an infant, or has a chronic health condition affected by water quality
- Whether your area has had repeated contamination issues or boil notices over the years
- Whether a landlord has dismissed a water quality concern without offering any testing or documentation

What to Check

- Whether your home's plumbing includes lead pipes, lead solder, or older fixtures, especially in homes built before 1986
- Whether your private well is located near a septic system, farm field, livestock area, or known industrial site

- Whether your local water utility or health department has published any contamination findings for your area
- What a basic bacteria test costs through your local health department, if you're on a well
- Whether your area has any known PFAS sources, such as a nearby military base or manufacturing site
- Whether your landlord has any water testing records, especially for lead, if you rent in an older building
- What your filter, if you have one, is actually certified to remove

What to Do Before Crisis

- If your home was built before 1986, find out whether lead testing is available through your water utility or health department
- If on a well, get a basic bacteria test done, especially if it has never been tested or wasn't tested when you moved in
- Look up whether your area has any documented PFAS, nitrate, or industrial contamination history
- Keep copies of any water testing results, notices, or official correspondence about water quality
- If pregnant or caring for an infant, ask specifically about nitrate and lead risk for your water source
- Write down the contact information for your local health department's environmental or water division

What Not to Waste Energy On

- Panicking over a word like "PFAS" or "lead" before finding out whether it actually applies to your specific home
- Accepting "it's probably fine" as an answer when no actual test has been done
- Buying an expensive filtration system before knowing what contaminant, if any, you're trying to remove
- Feeling guilty for not having tested your water sooner, when most people are never told they should
- Assuming a contamination problem found in your area decades ago has nothing to do with your water today
- Trying to personally investigate or prove a contamination source that should be the responsibility of a utility, landlord, or regulator

~5
Boil Notices

A notice goes up. Maybe it's a phone call from the city, maybe a text alert, maybe a flyer taped to the door, maybe just something a neighbor mentions in the hallway. The water in your area should be boiled before drinking, it says, until further notice. And then it stops, and you're left holding a dozen questions the notice didn't answer. Can the kids still take a bath? Is it safe to brush teeth with tap water? What about the coffee maker, the ice maker, the dog's water bowl, the formula you were about to mix? Is the dishwasher okay, or does that count as drinking water somehow? How long is "until further notice" actually going to be?

This chapter exists because boil water notices are one of the most common ways households are asked to interact with a water problem, and they are also one of the most poorly explained. The instructions are usually short, the timeline is usually vague, and the gap between what the notice says and what people actually need to know in their kitchen is often wide enough to cause real stress, especially for households managing infants, elders, or anyone with health vulnerabilities.

The first thing to understand is what a boil water notice is actually responding to. Most boil water notices are issued because of a biological concern: bacteria, viruses, or parasites that may have entered the water supply, usually because of a water main break, a drop in water pressure, a problem at the treatment plant, or flooding that affected the source water. Boiling water kills these organisms. That's what boiling does, and it's the whole reason boiling is the recommended response. A rolling boil for about a minute, generally a bit longer at high elevation, is enough to make the water safe from a biological standpoint.

What boiling does not do is remove chemicals, lead, or other contaminants that aren't biological. If a notice is about a chemical spill, industrial contamination, or something other than bacteria, boiling won't help and might even concentrate certain chemicals as the water evaporates. This is why it matters to read what kind of notice you actually received. A boil water notice is different from a "do not drink" notice, which usually means there's a chemical concern that boiling can't fix. It's also different from a "do not use" notice, which is the most serious version and usually means the water shouldn't be used for drinking, cooking, bathing, or even washing dishes, often because of a major chemical or fuel spill. Most notices people receive are boil water notices for biological concerns, but it's worth actually checking which type you've gotten, because the right response is different for each.

Assuming it's a standard boil water notice, here's how it breaks down in practical terms. Drinking water needs to be boiled, or you can use bottled water instead. This includes water for drinking directly, water used to make coffee or tea, water used to prepare foods that won't be cooked further, like a powdered drink mix or gelatin. Cooking water that will reach a boil anyway, like water for pasta or rice, is generally fine, because it's being boiled as part of cooking. Ice is a common blind spot:

ice made from tap water before the notice, or made from unboiled tap water during the notice, isn't safe, even though it's frozen. Frozen doesn't mean treated.

Brushing teeth is one of the most commonly asked questions, and the cautious answer is to use boiled or bottled water for this too, especially for young children who are more likely to swallow some water while brushing. Washing dishes by hand can be done with tap water, but dishes should either be allowed to air dry completely or be sanitized with a bleach solution, since residual water left on a dish could carry whatever the notice is concerned about. Dishwashers that have a sanitizing cycle with hot water are generally considered safe to use, though if you're uncertain, running an extra rinse or using the hot cycle specifically is a reasonable extra step.

Bathing and showering are usually fine for most healthy adults and older children, with the caution to avoid swallowing water and to be careful with infants, who are more likely to take in bath water. For infants, a sponge bath with boiled or bottled water is the more cautious choice during a notice.

Formula is one of the highest-stakes parts of a boil notice, because infants are one of the groups most vulnerable to the kind of contamination these notices are about. Formula that needs to be mixed with water should be mixed with water that has been boiled and then cooled, or with bottled water. This is one area where it's worth erring toward caution even if it feels like overkill, because the populations most at risk from a boil water notice are exactly the populations that formula feeding involves.

Pets often get left out of boil water notice instructions entirely, but the same logic generally applies. It's reasonable to give pets boiled or bottled water during a notice, particularly for smaller animals or animals with health issues, though most healthy adult pets aren't at the same level of risk as infants or immune-compromised people.

One of the things that makes boil water notices harder than they need to be is how unevenly they get communicated. In some areas, notices go out by text alert, email, and robocall all at once. In others, the only notification is a small item on a city website that most residents never check, or a notice mailed to a property owner who doesn't live there and doesn't pass it along to tenants. Apartment buildings are a particular weak point here. A landlord or property manager might receive a notice and either fail to pass it on to tenants, post it somewhere tenants don't see, or simply decide it isn't worth the effort. The same is true in workplaces, schools, and elder care facilities, where someone in a position of authority may know about a notice and not communicate it clearly to the people actually drinking the water.

If you're a renter and a boil water notice affects your building, it's worth documenting whether and how the notice was communicated to you, especially if it wasn't communicated promptly or at all. This matters less for the current notice, which you're dealing with regardless, and more for any future situation where a landlord's failure to communicate becomes part of a larger pattern that needs to be addressed.

When a boil water notice is lifted, there is still usually a small step between the official end of the notice and fully returning to normal. Many utilities recommend running cold water taps for a few minutes after the notice is lifted, because water may have been sitting in household pipes while the notice was in effect. That does not mean the danger is secretly continuing. It means the system needs to be cleared before everyone starts drinking from it again as if nothing happened.

It is also worth noticing whether a boil water notice is a one-time event or part of a pattern. A single notice after a storm, main break, or repair is not necessarily a sign that the whole water system is failing. Repeated notices in the same area are different, especially when the explanations are vague or there is no clear public answer about what is being fixed. Aging pipes, deferred maintenance, and underfunded utilities often do not fail all at once. They fail in a string of smaller interruptions, each treated like an isolated event until the pattern becomes too obvious to ignore. The goal is not to make a boil water notice feel bigger than it is. The goal is to know what the notice requires, what to do when it ends, and whether it is safe to brush your teeth without standing at the sink trying to figure it out from scratch.

Chapter 5 Action List: Boil Notices

What to Notice

- Whether a notice you've received is a boil water notice, a do not drink notice, or a do not use notice
- How the notice was communicated, and whether everyone in the household actually saw it
- Whether the notice gives a timeline, an end date, or only says "until further notice"
- Whether anyone in the household is pregnant, an infant, elderly, or immune-compromised
- Whether your building, workplace, or school has communicated the notice clearly
- Whether this is the first boil notice in your area recently, or one of several
- Whether ice, formula, or pet water has been addressed in your household's response

What to Check

- What type of notice you've received and what it actually requires
- Whether your household has any bottled water on hand, and how much
- Whether your stove or kettle works, in case boiling is needed
- Whether anyone in the household needs water for medical equipment, wound care, or medication
- Whether your landlord or building management has acknowledged the notice

- Whether your local utility's website explains when and how the notice will be lifted
- Whether any ice already in your freezer was made before or during the notice

What to Do Before Crisis

- Save your water utility's notification sign-up, if one exists, for future alerts
- Keep a small supply of bottled water on hand as a baseline, even when no notice is active
- Know how long your stove or kettle takes to bring water to a rolling boil
- Write down the boiling time recommended for your elevation, if you're at a higher elevation
- If you rely on formula, know in advance how you'd prepare it during a notice
- If renting, ask your landlord in advance how water notices are communicated to tenants

What Not to Waste Energy On

- Trying to interpret a vague notice without checking what type of notice it actually is
- Throwing out all the ice in your freezer in a panic before knowing whether it was made before the notice
- Assuming a single boil notice means your water system is permanently unsafe
- Feeling like you should have already known all of this before the notice arrived
- Blaming yourself if a landlord, school, or workplace failed to pass along a notice promptly

~6
Sewage

You flush the toilet and nothing happens the way it's supposed to. The water rises instead of disappearing, hovers near the rim for a second too long, and then slowly goes down, but slower than normal, with a sound that wasn't there before. A few minutes later, the tub in the bathroom down the hall starts to gurgle on its own, with no one running any water at all. By evening, there's a smell, faint at first, then unmistakable, coming from somewhere near the floor drain in the basement. Nobody wants to say the word out loud, but everyone in the house already knows what it probably is.

Sewage backup is one of those problems that carries a heavy layer of embarrassment on top of the actual issue, and that embarrassment makes everything worse. People delay calling for help because they're ashamed. They try to clean it up themselves without protection because admitting they need a professional feels like admitting something about themselves, rather than about a pipe. None of that shame belongs here. A sewage backup is not a referendum on how clean your house is or how well you manage your life. It's a plumbing and infrastructure failure, and it needs to be treated as the health issue it actually is.

To understand why these backups happen, it helps to know what the system is actually doing, in plain terms. Every toilet, sink, shower, and drain in your home connects to pipes that carry wastewater away from the house. In most homes connected to a municipal sewer system, those pipes eventually join a larger pipe, sometimes called a lateral, that runs from your house to the main sewer line under the street. From there, wastewater travels through the city's sewer system to a treatment plant, where it's processed before being released back into the environment, usually a river or other body of water, in a treated and safe form.

There's an important distinction between the sanitary sewer system, which carries wastewater from toilets, sinks, and drains, and the stormwater system, which carries rainwater from streets and roofs. In many older cities, these two systems are actually combined into a single set of pipes, which means that during heavy rain, the system can become overwhelmed with far more water than it was designed to handle all at once. When that happens, the excess has to go somewhere, and sometimes that somewhere is back up through the pipes into people's homes, usually through the lowest drain in the house, which is often a basement floor drain or a basement toilet.

This is one of the most important things to understand about sewage backups: they often aren't caused by anything you did. A backup that happens during or after heavy rain, especially if it happens to multiple homes on the same street at the same time, is almost always a sign of a system-wide problem, either a combined sewer overflow, a main line blockage, or a municipal pipe that's failing somewhere upstream of your house. You can have a perfectly maintained home and still get sewage backing up into your basement because of what's happening in pipes that belong to the city, not to you.

That said, backups can also be caused by something closer to home: a clog in your home's own lateral pipe, often from tree roots growing into an aging pipe and slowly blocking it, or from buildup that's accumulated over years. A single clogged toilet is usually a household-level problem. A backup affecting multiple fixtures at once, especially the lowest drains in the house, points toward something further down the line, either in your lateral or in the city's main.

Whatever the cause, the immediate priority is safety, not cleanup. Sewage contains bacteria, viruses, and parasites that can make people seriously ill, and contact with it should always involve protection: gloves at minimum, and ideally protective clothing and footwear that can be cleaned or discarded afterward. Children, elders, anyone with a compromised immune system, and pets should be kept away from the affected area entirely until it's been properly cleaned and disinfected. If the backup is significant, anything porous that came into contact with sewage, carpet, drywall, insulation, upholstered furniture, often can't be fully cleaned and may need to be removed and replaced. This isn't about being precious with belongings. It's about the fact that sewage-contaminated materials can continue to pose a health risk even after they look dry and clean.

If the backup is serious or affects multiple fixtures, the first call usually isn't to a plumber, it's to your local water or sewer department, or in some areas, a public works line specifically for sewer emergencies. Many municipalities have a number specifically for reporting sewer backups, and reporting it matters for two reasons. First, if the cause is on the city's side, they need to know, and your report may be one of several coming in that helps them locate a main line problem faster. Second, it creates a record. If this happens again, or if it's part of a pattern affecting your street, that record matters.

For homeowners, a sewage backup often becomes a question of insurance, and this is an area where a lot of people discover gaps they didn't know existed. Standard homeowners insurance policies frequently exclude sewer backup damage unless a specific endorsement, sometimes called sewer backup coverage or water backup coverage, has been added to the policy. If you've never specifically asked about this coverage, there's a real chance you don't have it, and finding that out during a backup, rather than before one, is one of the more painful ways to learn about an insurance gap.

For renters, a sewage backup raises the question of responsibility immediately, and the honest answer is that it depends, on your lease, on local law, and on whether the cause was something in the building's plumbing versus the city's main line. What doesn't depend on any of that is your right to have the situation addressed safely and promptly. A sewage backup that isn't cleaned up properly is a habitability issue, not a cosmetic one, and it's the kind of problem that justifies pushing harder than you might for something like a slow drain or a cosmetic repair. If a landlord is slow to respond, documenting everything, what happened, when, photos, any communication with the landlord, becomes important, both for getting the problem addressed and for any dispute that might follow about who's responsible for cleanup costs, lost belongings, or temporary living arrangements if the space becomes unusable.

One more thing worth knowing: a sewage smell without an obvious backup can sometimes mean something simpler, like a dry plumbing trap. The pipes under sinks, called P-traps, are designed to hold a small amount of water that blocks sewer gas from coming up into the house. If a drain hasn't been used in a while, like in a guest bathroom or a floor drain that rarely sees water, that trap can dry out, and sewer gas can start coming up through it. The fix for this is simple: pour some water down the drain to refill the trap. It's worth checking this before assuming a smell means a major backup, since it's one of the few sewage-related issues that's genuinely a quick, no-cost fix.

The bottom line with sewage is that it moves fast from inconvenience to health hazard, and the response needs to match that. Protect yourself and the people in your household first. Figure out whether this looks like a household-level problem or a city-level one, especially by paying attention to whether other homes nearby are affected. Call the right number, whether that's your sewer department, your landlord, or both. And document everything, because sewage problems have a way of becoming bigger conversations later, about insurance, about repairs, about responsibility, and the household that kept records is in a much stronger position than the one that just cleaned it up and tried to move on.

Chapter 6 Action List: Sewage

What to Notice

- A toilet that flushes slowly, gurgles, or causes other drains to bubble when used
- A sewage smell anywhere in the home, especially in the basement or near floor drains
- Multiple drains backing up at the same time, rather than just one fixture
- Backups that happen during or shortly after heavy rain
- Whether neighbors on your street have mentioned similar problems recently
- A persistent sewer gas smell coming from a drain that's rarely used
- Standing water or wastewater anywhere it shouldn't be, even in small amounts

What to Check

- Whether your homeowners insurance includes sewer or water backup coverage
- Whether your local water or sewer department has a specific number for reporting backups
- Whether your home's sewer lateral has a history of tree root or clogging issues
- Whether your lease specifies who is responsible for plumbing versus sewer line issues, if you rent
- Whether a rarely used drain in your home might just have a dry trap
- Whether your area has a combined sewer system, which can mean backups during heavy rain

- Whether any porous materials, carpet, drywall, furniture, have come into contact with a backup

What to Do Before Crisis

- Find out now whether your homeowners insurance covers sewer backups, and add coverage if it doesn't and you can
- Save your local sewer or public works emergency number somewhere accessible
- Keep a basic supply of gloves and cleaning materials for safely handling small sewage-related messes
- If you rent, find out in advance who you'd contact for a sewage backup and how quickly they typically respond
- Know where your home's main sewer cleanout is located, if it has one
- Run water periodically through rarely used drains to keep traps from drying out

What Not to Waste Energy On

- Feeling ashamed or embarrassed about a sewage backup, which is a plumbing issue, not a personal failing
- Cleaning up sewage-contaminated materials without gloves or protection
- Assuming a backup is automatically your fault before considering whether it's a city-wide issue
- Trying to save porous materials that came into contact with sewage rather than replacing them

- Delaying a call to your sewer department or landlord because the situation feels embarrassing to describe
- Assuming a sewage smell always means a major backup before checking for a simple dry trap

~7
Septic Systems

The drains in the house have been a little slow for weeks. Nobody mentioned it out loud, because slow drains are the kind of thing that's easy to live with until they're not. Then one morning the ground near the edge of the yard is soft in a way it shouldn't be, soft and a little sour smelling, even though it hasn't rained. A few days after that, an alarm starts going off somewhere near the basement stairs, a small electronic beep that nobody installed on purpose and nobody quite remembers being told about. Someone goes looking for paperwork: when was this last serviced, who did it, is there a number anywhere. There isn't. There's just a tank somewhere in the yard that has been quietly doing its job for years, and now it might not be.

For households on septic systems, which is most rural homes and a fair number of homes on the edges of small towns, this is one of the more common ways the system makes itself known: not with a dramatic failure, but with small signs that build until something forces the issue. And because septic systems are often misunderstood, even by the people whose homes depend on them, those small signs frequently get ignored for far too long.

A septic system is, at its core, a small, private wastewater treatment system that sits entirely on your property. Everything that goes down a drain in the house, from toilets, sinks, showers, and the washing machine, flows into a buried tank, usually made of concrete or plastic, located somewhere in the yard. Inside that tank, solids settle to the bottom, where bacteria break them down over time, while the liquid portion flows out into a drain field, sometimes called a leach field, which is a network of buried pipes that allow the liquid to slowly filter down through the soil. The soil itself does a lot of the final treatment work, filtering out remaining contaminants before the water rejoins the groundwater.

This system works well, for a long time, as long as a few things stay true. The tank needs to be pumped out periodically, because solids accumulate at the bottom and don't break down completely. How often depends on the size of the tank and how many people are using it, but a rough range for many households is every three to five years. The drain field needs functioning soil that can absorb liquid, which means it can be damaged by heavy vehicles driving over it, trees with roots that grow into the pipes, or simply by age, as the soil's ability to absorb water gradually decreases over decades of use. And the system needs to not be overwhelmed: too much water going in at once, whether from a household with more people than the system was designed for, or from a single day with multiple loads of laundry, long showers, and a dishwasher all running, can push more liquid into the drain field than it can handle.

Some septic systems include a pump, usually because the drain field is uphill from the tank or the property's layout requires it, and these systems often have an alarm that goes off if the pump isn't working or if liquid levels in the tank get too high. That alarm is not decorative. It's one of the few early warning systems a septic system has, and it should never be ignored or silenced without finding out what triggered it.

The warning signs of a septic system in trouble tend to show up gradually, then all at once. Slow drains throughout the house, not just one sink, are often an early sign, especially if plunging or snaking doesn't fix them for long. Gurgling sounds in pipes, especially after flushing or running water, can indicate the tank is full or the drain field isn't absorbing properly. A sewage smell, either inside the house near drains or outside near where the tank and drain field are located, is a sign that something is backing up or that the system isn't processing waste the way it should. And the most visible sign, soggy, spongy ground over the drain field, especially ground that stays wet or smells bad even when it hasn't rained, usually means the drain field has failed or is failing, and liquid that should be filtering into the soil is instead surfacing.

What goes into a septic system matters more than most people realize, because the system depends on bacteria to break down waste, and certain things disrupt that process or simply don't break down at all. Items that shouldn't go into a septic system include anything that doesn't biodegrade quickly: wipes of any kind, even ones labeled flushable, feminine hygiene products, paper towels, dental floss, cigarette butts, and cat litter. Grease and cooking oil poured down drains can solidify in pipes or the tank. Harsh chemicals, especially large amounts of bleach, drain cleaners, or antibacterial products, can kill off the bacteria the system depends on. And medications flushed down toilets don't just disappear, they pass through the system and can end up affecting the bacteria in the tank as well as the groundwater beyond it.

Water use matters too, in a way that's easy to overlook. A septic system is designed around an expected amount of water use, and anything that significantly exceeds that, a houseful of guests for a holiday, a broken toilet that's been running constantly, several loads of laundry done back to back, can temporarily overwhelm the drain field, especially if it's already aging or compromised. Spacing out heavy water use, and fixing running toilets or leaks promptly, isn't just about the water bill when you're on a septic system. It's about not pushing more into the system than the soil can handle.

Power outages affect septic systems with pumps in a specific way: if the pump can't run, wastewater can back up into the house rather than reaching the drain field, which means during an extended outage, a household with a pumped septic system needs to be conservative about water use, the same way a household on a well needs to think about water coming in.

The cost of septic failure is one of the hardest parts of this topic to talk about honestly, because it can be genuinely large. Pumping a tank typically costs a few hundred dollars. Repairing or replacing a failed drain field can cost many thousands, sometimes tens of thousands, depending on the size of the system, the soil conditions, and local regulations about how septic systems must be installed. For a household already stretched thin, the idea of a five-figure repair sitting somewhere underground, with no warning beyond a slow drain and a bad smell, is genuinely frightening. This is part of why pump-outs matter so much: a system that's pumped regularly and not abused tends to last for decades, while a system that's neglected can fail years before it should have, turning a maintenance cost into a replacement cost.

For renters, septic systems raise a question that does not come up with city sewer connections: who is responsible for maintenance, and does the landlord know the system's history. Many rental properties on septic have no clear record of when the tank was last pumped, because tenants come and go and landlords do not always track it. If you rent a home on septic, ask directly when the tank was last serviced. If the answer is "I don't know" or "not since we bought the place," that is useful information, not reassurance.

For anyone buying a home with a septic system, or anyone who has lived in one for years without thinking about it, the same questions apply: where is the tank, where is the drain field, when was it last pumped, and has it ever failed before. These questions do not require a specialist to ask. They require someone to ask them before the alarm goes off or the ground gets soft.

None of this is meant to make septic systems sound like ticking time bombs. Most septic systems, properly maintained, work quietly for decades, asking little beyond periodic pump-outs and reasonable care about what goes down the drain. The problem is not septic systems themselves. It is how often they are treated as invisible, exactly the kind of system nobody thinks about until they have no choice.

Chapter 7 Action List: Septic Systems

What to Notice

- Drains throughout the house that are slow, not just one isolated sink or toilet
- Gurgling sounds in pipes after flushing or running water
- A sewage smell inside the house near drains, or outside near the tank or drain field area
- Soggy, spongy, or smelly ground over the area where the tank or drain field is located
- Any alarm near the basement, utility area, or septic system that you don't recognize or have never heard before
- Multiple loads of laundry, long showers, or a full house of guests happening in a short period
- Whether you've ever flushed wipes, grease, or harsh chemicals down the drains

What to Check

- Where your septic tank and drain field are located on the property
- When the tank was last pumped, and by whom
- Whether your system has a pump and an alarm, and what the alarm is supposed to indicate
- Whether your lease or rental agreement says anything about septic maintenance responsibility, if you rent
- Whether any vehicles, equipment, or new structures have been placed over the drain field
- What size your tank is and roughly how often it should be pumped for your household size

- Whether your local health department keeps any records of septic permits or inspections for your property

What to Do Before Crisis

- Find out when your tank was last pumped, and schedule a pump-out if it's been more than three to five years or unknown
- Write down the location of your tank and drain field so it's not a guessing game later
- Stop putting wipes, grease, harsh chemicals, or medications down any drain in the house
- Fix any running toilets or dripping faucets promptly, since they add unnecessary load to the system
- During power outages, conserve water use if your system has a pump
- If renting, ask your landlord directly for the septic system's service history and put the request in writing

What Not to Waste Energy On

- Feeling embarrassed or ashamed about a septic problem, which is a maintenance and infrastructure issue, not a personal one
- Ignoring a septic alarm because it seems minor or you don't understand what it means
- Assuming a slow drain in one fixture is the same as a whole-system problem, or the reverse
- Ignoring the soggy ground over your drain field because it isn't currently causing a smell

- Ferrying water use around without addressing a known leak or running toilet
- Buying septic "treatment" additives as a substitute for an overdue pump-out

~8
Trash

The trash didn't come on Tuesday. By Wednesday, the bin at the curb is still full, and a couple of bags have been added to the top of it, because trash day comes every week whether or not anyone picks it up. By Thursday, something has gotten into one of those bags overnight, and now there's a mess on the lawn that someone has to clean up before the kids walk to the bus stop. Nobody got a notice. Nobody knows if it's a one-time thing, a holiday delay, or the start of something longer. The trash is just sitting there, becoming everyone's problem, one day at a time.

Trash removal is one of those systems that's so unremarkable when it works that most people couldn't tell you who runs it, how it's paid for, or what happens to anything after the truck pulls away. It's also one of the clearest examples of public health infrastructure hiding in plain sight. Garbage that sits too long attracts pests: rodents, insects, and in some areas, larger animals looking for an easy meal. Pests carry disease. Standing garbage in warm weather breeds bacteria and odors fast. None of this is dramatic until it is, and by the time it's dramatic, it's usually been building for a while.

In most places, trash service works one of a few ways. In many cities and suburbs, the local government either runs trash collection directly or contracts with a private hauling company, and residents pay for this service through taxes, a separate utility-style bill, or both. In some areas, especially unincorporated areas or smaller towns, residents contract individually with private haulers, meaning the household picks a company and pays them directly, with little oversight over pricing or service quality. And in many rural areas, there's no curbside pickup at all. Instead, households are responsible for taking their own trash to a transfer station or landfill, often on a schedule with specific hours, sometimes with a fee per load or a yearly permit.

Each of these systems has its own failure points. Municipal pickup can be affected by budget cuts, staffing shortages, or a hauling contract that changes hands, sometimes with little notice to residents about what's different. Private hauling in areas without much competition can mean steadily rising prices with no real alternative, since switching companies isn't always an option if there's only one operating in the area. And transfer stations and landfills, the rural option, depend on someone in the household having a working vehicle, the time to make the trip, and the ability to pay whatever fee applies, which turns trash disposal into a transportation and scheduling problem on top of everything else.

When trash service is reduced, privatized further, or becomes too expensive for a household to keep up with, the consequences show up fast, because trash doesn't pause itself while people figure things out. A household that falls behind on payments to a private hauler may simply stop having pickup, with garbage accumulating until either the bill gets paid or someone finds another way to get rid of it. In apartment buildings, the consequences are often shared rather than individual: a dumpster that isn't emptied often enough becomes a problem for every unit in the building, regardless of how careful any individual tenant is, and tenants often have no direct relationship with whoever is responsible for that dumpster's service schedule.

This is where the household-level work tends to land, and it tends to land on whoever is paying the closest attention to the kitchen, the yard, and the kids. Someone notices the smell first. Someone decides whether it's safe to let a toddler play in the yard if there's been an issue with pests near uncollected trash. Someone figures out where the nearest dumpster, transfer station, or alternative disposal option is, if the regular system breaks down even temporarily. Someone deals with the aftermath when an animal gets into the bags. This is unglamorous, easily dismissed work, and it's also genuinely connected to keeping a household healthy.

Separate from regular household trash, there's a category of waste that requires different handling, and most households have more of it sitting around than they realize: hazardous household waste. This includes things like old paint and paint thinner, motor oil, car batteries and household batteries, pesticides and herbicides, cleaning chemicals, fluorescent bulbs, and electronics like old phones, laptops, and televisions. It also includes medications, particularly ones that shouldn't be flushed or thrown in regular trash because of how they can affect water systems or be accessed by others, and in some households, used needles or other medical sharps.

None of these things belong in a regular trash bag, and most communities have specific drop-off programs, collection events, or designated facilities for hazardous waste, electronics, and medications, often free or low-cost. The problem is that almost nobody knows this until they're standing in their garage with a can of old paint, wondering whether it's okay to just put it out with everything else. The honest answer is usually no, but the information about what to do instead is often buried on a county or city website that most people have never had a reason to visit.

Storm debris and disaster cleanup add another layer entirely. After a major storm, flood, or other event that generates a large amount of debris all at once, fallen branches, damaged furniture, ruined drywall, regular trash pickup is often suspended or overwhelmed, and many areas set up separate debris collection schedules or drop-off points specifically for storm-related waste. Knowing that this distinction exists, and that storm debris often needs to be separated from regular trash and placed in a specific way to be collected, can save a household from putting debris out incorrectly and having it sit for weeks because it didn't match what the regular trucks are equipped to handle.

Illegal dumping is a problem that affects rural areas and lower-income neighborhoods disproportionately, and it's worth naming as exactly what it is: a symptom of inadequate, inaccessible, or unaffordable legitimate disposal options. When transfer stations are far away, have limited hours, or charge fees that some households can't afford, and when there's no curbside alternative, some amount of trash ends up dumped along rural roads, in ditches, or on vacant land. This isn't a moral failing unique to whoever does the dumping. It's what happens when a system makes legitimate disposal genuinely difficult for some portion of the population, and the consequences, an ugly roadside, contaminated runoff, an eyesore that depresses property values, land on everyone nearby regardless of who's responsible.

Recycling deserves a brief, honest mention, mostly because of how much confusion surrounds it. Recycling programs vary enormously by location in terms of what's actually accepted, and "recyclable" symbols on packaging don't guarantee that an item will actually be recycled in your area, or anywhere. Some materials that seem recyclable are routinely rejected by local programs because there's no market for them, or because they're contaminated by other materials mixed in with them. None of this means recycling is pointless, but it does mean that treating recycling as a solution to a household's waste volume, or as something that erases the impact of consumption, is mostly a comforting story rather than an accurate one. Knowing what your specific local program actually takes, and not wishfully tossing things into the bin that don't belong there, is more useful than assuming the system will sort it out.

For most households, the practical reality of trash is this: it's a weekly or near-weekly task that depends on a system most people never think about, until that system slows down, gets more expensive, or simply stops, at which point it becomes urgent very quickly, because garbage doesn't wait politely while anyone figures out what to do next.

Chapter 8 Action List: Trash

What to Notice

- Whether trash, recycling, or yard waste pickup has been missed, delayed, or changed recently without explanation
- Pests, animals, or unusual smells around trash storage areas, indoors or outside
- Whether a shared dumpster, if you live in an apartment, seems to be emptied less often than it used to be
- Hazardous items accumulating in the garage, closet, or under the sink, such as old paint, batteries, or chemicals
- Unused or expired medications that have been sitting around without a plan for disposal
- Whether your area has had any storm debris or disaster cleanup needs recently
- Roadside dumping or illegal dumping becoming more common in your area

What to Check

- Whether your trash service is run by the local government, a private hauler, or requires self-haul to a transfer station
- Your local hazardous waste, electronics, and medication disposal programs and where they're located
- Whether your area has a specific protocol for storm debris separate from regular trash

- What your local recycling program actually accepts, rather than assuming based on packaging symbols
- If you live in an apartment, who is responsible for the dumpster's service schedule
- Whether there's a fee schedule for transfer station or landfill use in your area, if that's your only option
- Whether your trash hauler has had any service complaints or changes reported locally

What to Do Before Crisis

- Write down your trash pickup day, hauler name, and a contact number for missed pickups
- Find your nearest hazardous waste or electronics drop-off location and its hours
- Set a date to clear out old paint, batteries, chemicals, and electronics that have been sitting unused
- Find out how your area handles medication disposal, including any take-back programs at pharmacies
- If self-hauling, know the location, hours, and fees for your nearest transfer station before you need it
- If in an apartment, find out who manages the dumpster and how to report it if it's consistently overflowing

What Not to Waste Energy On

- Feeling responsible for a missed pickup that's a service-wide issue rather than something specific to your household
- Assuming a recycling symbol on packaging means an item will actually be recycled in your area
- Holding onto hazardous waste indefinitely out of uncertainty about disposal, rather than looking up the local program
- Blaming yourself or neighbors for illegal dumping caused by inadequate disposal access in the area
- Treating a shared dumpster problem in an apartment building as something only you can fix
- Trying to handle large storm debris cleanup entirely on your own before checking what local programs exist

~9
Flooding & Mold

It rains for two days straight, the kind of steady rain that doesn't look dramatic from inside but doesn't stop either. On the third morning, someone goes down to the basement for laundry and stops at the bottom of the stairs, because the floor is wet, not flooded exactly, but wet in a way that wasn't true yesterday. There's a thin sheen of water spreading from one corner, and along the wall near the floor, a stain that's been there for a while but looks darker now, with a smell that's hard to place but unmistakably not right. Outside, the storm drain at the end of the driveway is gurgling under a small lake that's formed where the yard slopes down toward the road.

Water in places it doesn't belong is one of the most common household problems there is, and it's also one of the most consistently minimized, both by the people living with it and by the landlords, insurers, and contractors they have to deal with afterward. Part of the reason is that water damage often doesn't look like an emergency. There's no flush, no smell of sewage, no immediate health symptom. There's just dampness, and dampness is the kind of thing that's easy to put off dealing with, right up until it isn't.

To understand why basements flood, it helps to think about where water goes when it falls from the sky. Rain that lands on a roof is supposed to be channeled by gutters and downspouts away from the foundation of the house. Rain that lands on the ground is supposed to either soak into the soil or run off toward a drainage system, whether that's a storm drain, a ditch, a culvert, or simply a slope that directs water away from buildings. When any part of this system fails, whether it's a clogged gutter, a downspout that empties right next to the foundation instead of away from it, ground that's sloped toward the house instead of away from it, or a storm drain system that's undersized or blocked, water ends up somewhere it shouldn't, and basements and crawlspaces, being the lowest points of most homes, are usually where it ends up first.

Sump pumps exist specifically to deal with this. A sump pump sits in a small pit, usually in a basement or crawlspace, and its job is to pump groundwater or seepage out and away from the house before it can accumulate. A sump pump that's working is invisible, just an occasional hum from somewhere in the basement. A sump pump that isn't working, whether because it's broken, because it's not plugged in, or because the power is out, means that water that would normally be pumped away simply stays, and basements that have never flooded before can flood for the first time the moment that pump stops running.

This is one of the more important overlaps in this book: power outages and flooding aren't separate problems. A storm severe enough to cause flooding is often also severe enough to cause power outages, which means the exact moment a sump pump is most needed is often the exact moment it can't run, unless it's connected to a battery backup. This is worth knowing not to create more anxiety, but because it explains why some households that have never had basement water issues suddenly do, during a storm that knocks out power for several hours.

Stormwater systems themselves are public infrastructure, and like other infrastructure in this book, they age, get overwhelmed, and don't always get the maintenance or upgrades they need. Many older neighborhoods have stormwater systems that were designed decades ago, for rainfall patterns that don't match what's happening now. When a storm drops more rain in an hour than the system was built to handle, water backs up, pools in streets, and finds its way into the lowest points it can reach, which sometimes means basements connected to that same overwhelmed system. A flooded basement during a major storm, especially one affecting multiple homes on the same street, often isn't a sign that anything is specifically wrong with your house. It's a sign that the public system serving your whole area wasn't built for the amount of water it's now being asked to handle.

Once water is in a basement or crawlspace, the clock on mold starts immediately, and this is the part of flooding that causes the most lasting damage, often far more than the water itself. Mold needs moisture and time, and it doesn't need much of either. Materials that stay wet for more than about a day or two, carpet, drywall, insulation, wood framing, can begin growing mold within that window, and once mold has established itself inside a wall or under flooring, it can be extremely difficult to fully remove without tearing out the affected materials.

Mold is a health issue, not just a property issue, and it's worth being direct about that. For people with asthma or other respiratory conditions, mold exposure can trigger or worsen symptoms significantly. Children's developing respiratory systems can be more affected by mold than adults'. People with weakened immune systems can face more serious health effects from certain types of mold. And for anyone living with ongoing, unaddressed mold, even without a dramatic reaction, there's a kind of background health cost that doesn't always get connected back to its source, especially if the mold is hidden behind a wall or under flooring where nobody's actually looking at it.

For renters, water intrusion and mold sit at the center of one of the most common landlord disputes there is, and the dynamics are predictable. A leak or flooding event happens. The tenant reports it. The landlord, if they respond at all, may send someone to mop up visible water without addressing the underlying cause, whether that's a roof issue, a drainage problem, or a foundation crack. The visible water goes away, the tenant is told it's handled, and weeks or months later, mold appears, sometimes visibly, sometimes only as a smell or as health symptoms that nobody connects to the apartment until someone mentions it feels better when they're not home. By that point, the original water event may not even be in anyone's memory as connected to the mold that's showing up now.

This is why documentation matters so much with water intrusion specifically, more than with almost any other issue in this book. Photos of water when it happens, dated, with a note about where it came from if that's known. Written notice to a landlord, even if a phone call happened first, because phone calls don't leave records. Any response from the landlord, in writing if possible. And later, if mold appears, photos of that too, with the same kind of dating and description. A renter who can show "water came in here on this date, I reported it, here's what happened, and now there's mold in the same spot" is in a fundamentally different position than a renter who can only say "there's mold and I don't really know how long it's been there."

Insurance is its own complicated piece of this, and the short version is that standard homeowners insurance often treats different types of water damage very differently. Water that suddenly comes from inside the home, a burst pipe, for instance, is often covered. Water that comes from outside the home, flooding from rain, groundwater, or a body of water, is often not covered by a standard policy at all, and requires separate flood insurance, which many homeowners don't have, especially if they're not in an officially designated flood zone, even though flooding can and does happen outside those zones.

Road flooding deserves a mention here too, because it's connected to the same drainage systems and can isolate a household just as effectively as flooding inside a home. A road that floods during heavy rain, even briefly, can cut off access to a home for hours, which matters enormously if someone needs to get to work, to a pharmacy, to a medical appointment, or if an ambulance would need to reach the house in an emergency. Knowing which roads near you flood, and how often, is part of understanding your household's actual exposure to water-related infrastructure problems, even if the water never touches your house directly.

None of this is meant to suggest that every damp basement is a crisis, or that every household needs to live in fear of the next storm. Most water intrusion, caught early and dried out quickly, doesn't turn into a major mold problem. What matters is catching it early, understanding why it happened, whether that's a household-level issue like a gutter or sump pump, or a larger drainage and infrastructure issue affecting the whole area, and not letting "it's just a little damp" turn into months of unaddressed moisture sitting quietly behind a wall.

Chapter 9 Action List: Flooding & Mold

What to Notice

- Damp spots, standing water, or wet flooring in a basement or crawlspace, even small amounts
- Musty smells anywhere in the home, especially in basements, closets, or behind furniture
- Visible mold growth on walls, ceilings, around windows, or on stored items
- Whether gutters are clogged or downspouts empty close to the foundation
- Whether the ground around your home slopes toward or away from the house
- Whether any roads near you flood during heavy rain, and how often
- Whether anyone in the household has asthma, allergies, or respiratory symptoms that seem worse at home

What to Check

- Whether your home has a sump pump, and if so, whether it's plugged in and working
- Whether your sump pump has a battery backup for use during power outages
- When your gutters were last cleaned and whether downspouts direct water away from the foundation
- Whether your homeowners insurance covers water backup or flood damage, or whether you need separate flood insurance

- Whether your home is in a designated flood zone, and what that does and doesn't mean for risk
- Any past water intrusion events in your home, even minor ones, and what was done about them
- Whether your lease specifies anything about reporting leaks or water damage, if you rent

What to Do Before Crisis

- Test your sump pump, if you have one, and consider a battery backup if you don't already have one
- Clean gutters and check that downspouts direct water at least several feet away from the foundation
- Photograph and document any existing water stains, damp areas, or musty smells now, before they become bigger problems
- Find out whether your homeowners insurance covers flooding, and look into flood insurance if it doesn't
- If renting, report any signs of water intrusion in writing, even minor ones, and keep a copy
- Identify which roads near your home are prone to flooding and what alternate routes exist

What Not to Waste Energy On

- Assuming a small damp spot will dry out on its own without checking why it's happening
- Cleaning up visible mold without addressing the moisture source that caused it

- Believing "it's not a flood zone" means flooding can't happen to your home
- Feeling like water intrusion reflects poorly on how you keep your home
- Waiting to document a leak or flood until it becomes a bigger, harder-to-prove problem
- Assuming a landlord's quick mop-up means the underlying issue has actually been fixed

~10
The EATMS Water & Waste Plan

By now, the pieces are mostly on the table. You know more than you did about where your water comes from and where your waste goes, what a boil notice actually requires, what contamination looks like and doesn't look like, what a septic alarm means, why the trash matters more than it seems, and how quickly a damp basement can become a much bigger problem. None of that knowledge fixes anything by itself. What it does is turn a long list of vague worries into a shorter list of specific things, and specific things can be planned for in a way that vague worries can't.

This chapter is about putting those specific things together into something usable. Not a binder full of forms, that's what the Supplemental Section is for, but a way of thinking that you can carry with you, into a new home, a new lease, a conversation with a landlord, or just an ordinary Tuesday when something starts to go wrong.

The foundation of a water and waste plan is knowing your household's basic map: where water comes in, and where waste goes out. This sounds simple, and for some households it is, but for a surprising number of people, these are questions they've never actually answered, because they've never needed to until the day they suddenly did. If you're on municipal water, do you know which utility serves you, and do you know how to find their notices and reports? If you're on a well, do you know where it is, how old the pump is, and when it was last tested? If your waste goes to a sewer, do you know whether your home has had backup issues before, and whether your insurance covers them? If you're on a septic system, do you know where the tank and drain field are, and when it was last pumped? These aren't trick questions, and you don't need to know the answers from memory. What matters is knowing that these are the right questions, and having a place where the answers live once you find them.

From that foundation, the next layer is knowing your household's specific vulnerabilities, the things that make a given problem more or less urgent for the people actually living in your home. A boil water notice is a different event in a household with an infant who needs formula than in a household of healthy adults. A sewer backup is a different event for a renter than a homeowner with the right insurance. A power outage that stops a well pump or a septic pump is a different event for a household on a well or pumped septic system than for a household on municipal water and sewer. None of this is about ranking whose situation is worse. It's about being honest with yourself about which chapters in this book matter most for your specific household, right now, so that if you only have time and energy to prepare for a few things, you're preparing for the right few things.

The next layer is warning signs, and this is where the chapters in this book really earn their place in a plan. Slow drains, strange tastes or smells, a septic alarm, a damp basement, a rising water bill, repeated notices from your utility: each of these is a small signal, and small signals are useful precisely because they show up before the big failure does. A household that's been paying attention to small signals isn't surprised in the same way by the big one. They've already started a conversation with a landlord, or scheduled a pump-out, or found out where the local hazardous waste drop-off is, before any of it became urgent. This is the heart of what "before crisis" means throughout this book: not predicting the future, just not waiting for the worst version of the problem before doing anything.

Documentation is the thread that runs through almost every chapter, and it's worth saying clearly why it matters so much in this particular area of life. Water and waste problems are uniquely prone to becoming "he said, she said" situations: a landlord who says a leak was fixed, a utility that says a notice was sent, an insurer who says a claim wasn't filed in time. In almost every one of these situations, the household with dates, photos, and written records is in a stronger position than the household that has only memory and frustration. This isn't about preparing for conflict before it exists. It's about not being caught without proof on the day proof suddenly matters.

Emergency water storage deserves a realistic place in this plan, neither ignored nor turned into its own anxiety. A small amount of stored drinking water, enough for a day or two for everyone in the household, including pets, is genuinely useful during a boil notice, a contamination event, or a short-term outage that affects a well pump. It doesn't need to be elaborate, and it doesn't need to be more than your space and budget comfortably allow. The goal is a buffer, not a bunker. If you have the space for more, more doesn't hurt. If you don't, a few days' worth is still meaningfully better than none, and none is the situation most households are actually in.

Hygiene and toilets during disruption are worth thinking through in advance, because this is one of the areas where people tend to freeze up the most when something actually happens. If water is unsafe or unavailable, or if a toilet can't be used because of a sewer or septic problem, what's the household's actual plan? For most people, the honest answer involves things like: using stored or bottled water for hand washing and basic hygiene, knowing whether there's a safe alternative toilet option nearby, like a neighbor, a workplace, or a public building, and understanding that this is a short-term bridge, not a long-term solution. Thinking about this for five minutes before it happens is enormously more useful than thinking about it for the first time while it's happening.

Your contact list is one of the simplest and most underused tools available, and it belongs in this plan even though the actual list lives in the Supplemental Section. The contacts that matter most are the ones you're least likely to remember correctly under stress: your water utility's emergency line, your sewer or public works department, your septic service company if you have one, your local health department, and, if you rent, your landlord's actual responsive contact information, not just the one on the lease that goes to voicemail. Having these written down somewhere accessible, not just saved in a phone that might be dead, is a small thing that consistently makes a real difference.

Finally, this plan has to include an honest accounting of what's beyond your household's control, because pretending otherwise is where a lot of unnecessary stress comes from. You cannot personally fix aging water mains, cannot personally regulate PFAS, cannot personally force a landlord to respond faster than they're willing to, and cannot personally prevent a storm from overwhelming a stormwater system that was undersized before you ever moved in. What you can do is notice problems early, document them clearly, know who's actually responsible for what, and make the decisions that are genuinely yours to make, about your own household's water storage, your own documentation, your own response to a notice or a smell or a bill that doesn't add up.

That's the whole plan, really. Not a guarantee that nothing will go wrong, because something eventually will, in every home, sooner or later. But a household that knows its water source, knows its waste system, watches for the signs that matter, keeps a record when something happens, and knows who to call, is a household that moves through these problems instead of being flattened by them. That's not nothing. For most people, most of the time, that's exactly enough.

Chapter 10 Action List: The EATMS Water Plan

What to Notice

- Whether you've actually identified your household's water source and waste system, or whether that's still an open question
- Which water or waste problem in this book felt most relevant to your specific household
- Whether anyone in your home has needs that would make a water or waste disruption more urgent
- Whether you've been ignoring any small warning sign because it hasn't become a big problem yet
- Whether you have any documentation at all of past water, sewage, or drainage issues
- Whether your emergency contacts are written down anywhere besides your phone
- Whether your household has ever talked through what you'd actually do during a boil notice or toilet outage

What to Check

- Your water source and whether it's municipal or a private well
- Whether your home is on sewer or septic, and the basic condition of that system
- Your most recent water bill for any unexplained changes
- Whether your homeowners or renters insurance covers water backup or flooding

- Whether your landlord, if you have one, has a record of past water or plumbing issues
- What your household would actually do for drinking water and toilet use during a multi-day disruption
- Whether your local utility, health department, and public works numbers are saved anywhere accessible

What to Do Before Crisis

- Write down your household's water source, waste system, and the basics of both in one place
- Identify the one or two water and waste risks most relevant to your household and address those first
- Start a simple written record for any future leaks, odors, notices, or drainage issues, with dates and photos
- Store a small, realistic amount of drinking water for your household, including pets
- Build a short contact list for your utility, sewer or septic service, health department, and landlord if applicable
- Walk through, even briefly, what your household would do if the toilet or tap water were unusable for a day

What Not to Waste Energy On

- Trying to build a plan that covers every possible scenario before you've covered the most likely ones

- Feeling like you should have already done all of this before reading the book
- Comparing your household's preparation to someone with more money, space, or homeownership
- Treating this plan as something that needs to be finished perfectly in one sitting
- Worrying about problems that belong to a utility, landlord, or local government as if they were yours to solve
- Letting the size of the larger systems in this book make your own small, concrete steps feel pointless

Conclusion

This book also started inside the house. The tap that suddenly tasted wrong. The toilet that wouldn't flush right. The boil water notice on the door. The basement floor that stayed wet a little too long. The trash that didn't come, the septic alarm nobody had heard before, the bill that crept up without explanation. None of these are dramatic openings, but they're honest ones, because this is where water and waste failure actually shows up: not as a headline, but as a problem inside a specific home, usually noticed first by whoever is paying closest attention to that home, and usually left for that same person to figure out.

The systems behind those moments are old, large, and mostly invisible until something goes wrong. Pipes laid decades before anyone currently living in a house was born. Treatment plants and sewer mains that depend on funding decisions made far away and long ago. Wells and septic systems that sit quietly on private property with no one checking on them unless someone thinks to ask. None of it was built with a particular household in mind, and none of it adjusts itself based on who's most affected when it fails: the renter with no authority over the pipes, the household on a private well with no testing budget, the family already stretched thin before a sewage backup or a flooded basement adds a new expense nobody planned for.

Knowing where responsibility actually sits matters here just as much as it did with power and heat. The renter dealing with a sewage backup did not cause the aging sewer main that overflowed during a storm. The household drinking from a well with lead-contaminated water did not install the pipes that put it there, sometimes decades before they ever moved in. The family facing a five-figure septic repair did not create the soil conditions or the system's age, and the household whose water bill keeps climbing did not vote to privatize the utility that's now billing them. In each case, the household lives with the consequence. The household did not create the cause.

What a household can do is real, and this book has tried to make that as concrete as possible. Know your water source and your waste system. Pay attention to the small signs before they become big ones. Keep records, because records are what turn a vague complaint into something a landlord, a utility, or an insurer has to actually respond to. Store a little water, know your contacts, and have at least a rough idea of what you'd do if the tap or the toilet stopped working tomorrow. None of that is nothing. But none of it replaces aging pipes, funds a treatment plant upgrade, regulates a chemical, or forces a landlord to act faster than they're willing to. That work belongs to utilities, regulators, landlords, and the public decisions that shape what they're required to do.

Water and waste are not background conveniences. They are where public neglect, private cost, and household labor all meet, often in the most literal sense, in a basement, a bathroom, or a glass of water that used to be something nobody thought about. You already knew that, every time you smelled something wrong, worried about a bill, or wondered whether the water was actually safe. This book tried to tell you what was actually happening behind that knowledge, and to give you a clearer sense of what's yours to handle and what never should have been.

Addendum: AI, Data Centers, & Water Strain

There's a part of the water story that doesn't show up on a household bill directly, at least not yet in most places, but it's worth understanding, because it's one of the clearest examples of how a household's water security can be shaped by decisions that have nothing to do with the household at all.

Large data centers, the buildings full of servers that power everything from cloud storage to streaming video to artificial intelligence systems, use enormous amounts of water. Much of it goes toward cooling. Servers generate heat constantly, and many data centers use water-based cooling systems, sometimes evaporative systems that lose water to the air the way a swamp cooler does, because it's often cheaper than other cooling methods. A single large data center can use as much water in a day as a small town.

As AI systems have expanded rapidly, the number of new data centers being built, and the size of each one, has grown along with them. These facilities are often built near sources of cheap land, available power, and, importantly, available water, which has meant a growing number of them are located in places that are already dealing with water stress: parts of the country experiencing drought, areas with aquifers that are already being drawn down faster than they recharge, and communities where municipal water systems are already stretched.

When a data center moves into an area, it becomes a new, large user of the same water system everyone else depends on. In some cases, this has led to direct conflict: communities raising concerns about whether a new data center's water use will affect their own water pressure, well levels, or future water availability, while companies and local governments, eager for the tax revenue and jobs a data center can bring, sometimes negotiate water access agreements with limited public input or transparency about how much water is actually involved.

This connects back to almost everything else in this book. A community with aging water infrastructure, a treatment plant near capacity, or groundwater already under stress has less room to absorb a large new user without affecting pressure, cost, or long-term availability. And because data centers are often presented as economic development, decisions about them can move quickly, sometimes faster than the public conversation about their water impact.

None of this means every data center is draining every nearby town dry, or that households should panic about a new facility nearby. It means water, like power, is a shared and finite local resource, and large new users are a legitimate thing for communities to ask about, the same way they might ask about roads, schools, or sewer capacity. If a data center is proposed or built near you, questions about its water source, its water use, and whether that use was included in local water planning are reasonable questions, not fringe ones. They are easier to ask before a facility is built than after.

Supplemental Section

The materials here are meant to be used, not just read. Copy them, fill them in, print them out, or work through them on a notes page. They support the chapters but do not replace them. Start with whatever is most urgent for your household and come back to the rest.

1. Household Water Source Checklist

Fill in the following for your home:

• Water source: municipal, private well, or community/shared system
• Utility name or well location:
• Account number, if applicable:
• Filter type, if any, and what it's certified to remove:
• Date filter cartridge was last changed:
• Main water shutoff valve location:
• Most recent water quality report date, if on municipal water:
• Most recent well test date and what it tested for, if applicable:
• Landlord or property manager contact, if renting:

2. Well Household Checklist

Write in the following if your home is on a private well:

• Pump type and approximate age:

- Pressure tank location:
- Treatment system, if any, and what it does:
- Last test date and results:
- Last service date:
- Does the household have a plan for water during a power outage: yes or no
- Known issues or repairs needed:

3. Municipal Water Checklist

Fill in the following if your home is on municipal water:

- Utility name and account number:
- Customer service number:
- Emergency or main-break reporting number:
- Where to find local notices: website, text alert, or mailing
- Most recent water quality report reviewed: yes or no
- Known lead service line status for your address or block:
- Sign-up status for outage or notice alerts: enrolled or not enrolled

4. Water Warning Signs Log

Keep a separate entry for each incident, recording the following in order:

1. Date
2. What was noticed: smell, taste, color, pressure, or sediment
3. Where in the home

4. Any illness or symptoms in the household
5. Photos taken: yes or no
6. Who was contacted: utility, landlord, or health department
7. Response received
8. Resolution date

A pattern across several entries is worth more than any single one.

5. Water Testing Notes

When deciding whether to test, consider testing:

• After moving in
• After any nearby construction or land disturbance
• If anyone in the household is pregnant or has an infant
• If the home was built before 1986
• If any warning sign from this book appears

What to ask for: bacteria, lead, nitrates, or a broader panel depending on local concerns Where to send a sample: local health department or certified lab

Approximate cost:
Where results are kept:
Date of most recent test:

6. Boil Notice Response Sheet

When a notice arrives, fill in the following:

• Notice received date:
• Type of notice: boil water, do not drink, or do not use
• How the notice was communicated:
• End date, or whether it says "until further notice":

Then work through this checklist:

1. Drinking and cooking water plan
2. Ice plan: discard ice made before or during the notice
3. Formula or infant feeding plan
4. Tooth brushing plan
5. Dish washing plan
6. Bathing plan, especially for infants
7. Pet water plan

Notice lifted date: Post-notice flush completed: yes or no

7. Emergency Water Planning Page

• Minimum drinking water target: number of people times one gallon per day, for at least two days
• Hygiene water needs:
• Pets and their water needs:
• Anyone needing water for medication, formula, or medical equipment:
• Current storage amount:
• Storage location:
• Rotation or replacement date:

This is a buffer, not a bunker.

8. Sewer Backup Checklist

When a backup happens, work through these in order:

1. Note the date and time
2. Identify what happened and where it appeared
3. Take photos
4. Take safety steps, including gloves and keeping people and pets away
5. Contact the sewer department, landlord, or plumber
6. Record any reference or report number
7. Note whether other homes nearby were affected
8. Contact insurance if applicable

Cleanup and repair notes:

9. Septic System Record Page

- Tank location:
- Drain field location:
- Tank size, if known:
- Last pump-out date and company:
- Last inspection date:
- Alarm present: yes or no, and what it indicates
- Do-not-flush list reviewed with household: yes or no
- Known issues or repairs needed:

A working system asks very little. Pay attention now, so it doesn't ask more later.

10. Household Drain and Toilet Warning List

For each fixture, note any of the following: slow draining, gurgling, repeated clogs, odor, or recent backup.

- Kitchen sink:
- Bathroom sink or sinks:
- Tub or shower:
- Toilet or toilets:
- Basement or floor drain:
- Washing machine drain:
- Any rarely used drain that may need water added to its trap:

11. Trash and Hazardous Waste Map

- Regular pickup day and hauler:
- Missed pickup contact number:
- Nearest transfer station or landfill, hours, and fees:
- Hazardous waste drop-off location and hours:
- Electronics recycling location:
- Medication take-back location:
- Battery and bulb disposal location:
- What your local recycling program actually accepts:
- Storm debris protocol, if known:

12. Flooding and Mold Documentation Log

Keep a separate entry for each incident.

1. Date

2. Location in home
3. Photos taken: yes or no
4. Smell or visible mold present: yes or no
5. Suspected source of water
6. Landlord notified: yes or no, date and method
7. Insurance claim filed: yes or no
8. Repairs attempted and by whom
9. Follow-up needed
10. Local Contacts Page

Fill this in before anything goes wrong:

• Water utility: name, customer service number, emergency line
• Sewer or public works department: name and number
• Local health department, environmental division:
• Septic service company:
• Plumber:
• Trash hauler or transfer station:
• Code enforcement:
• Landlord or property manager: name, number, preferred contact method
• Emergency management:
• Neighbor one: name and number
• Neighbor two: name and number

14. What Not to Buy in Panic

After a bad water or sewage event, panic spending feels like the answer. It usually is not. Before spending money, read this list.

• A whole-house filtration system before knowing what, if anything, is actually in your water. Test first, filter second.
• Large amounts of bottled water as a long-term strategy. It's useful short-term, but expensive, heavy, and impractical long-term.
• Septic tank additives as a substitute for an overdue pump-out. They don't replace mechanical service.
• Expensive emergency toilets or sanitation kits before understanding your actual backup options, including neighbors, workplaces, or nearby public buildings.
• Chemical test kits for contaminants you have no specific reason to suspect. A targeted test from a real lab is more useful than a broad kit that may not be reliable.

The most useful preparations are almost always inexpensive: a written record of your water source and waste system, a small water supply, and a list of who to call.

15. What to Do This Week

Start here. These actions cost nothing or very little and make a real difference.

1. Find out whether your home is on municipal water or a private well, and whether it's on sewer or septic.
2. Locate your main water shutoff valve.
3. If on a well, find out when it was last tested and for what.
4. If on municipal water, find and review your most recent water quality report.

5. Write down your local water utility, sewer department, and health department contact information.
6. Start a simple log for any current or past water, drain, or drainage issues, with dates and photos.
7. Store a small amount of drinking water if you don't already have any on hand.
8. Fill in at least the utility numbers and landlord contact on the Local Contacts Page.

Suggested Reading, Watching, & Listening

The resources listed here extend the ideas in this book without requiring a background in engineering, hydrology, or environmental policy. They are organized by format and theme. Start with what matches the current household situation or the chapter that felt most urgent.

On Water Systems and Infrastructure

The Big Thirst: The Secret Life and Turbulent Future of Water by Charles Fishman is a readable look at how water systems actually work, why they're taken for granted, and what happens when they start to fail. It connects directly to the chapters on drinking water, wells, and municipal systems.

Water 4.0: The Past, Present, and Future of the World's Most Vital Resource by David Sedlak covers the history of water treatment and distribution in plain terms, with attention to why so much American water infrastructure is aging and what it would take to modernize it.

The Environmental Working Group maintains a searchable national database of municipal water quality reports at ewg.org, often easier to navigate than a utility's own consumer confidence report.

On Contamination, Lead, and Environmental Health

What the Eyes Don't See: A Story of Crisis, Resistance, and Hope in an American City by Mona Hanna-Attisha is written by the pediatrician who helped expose the Flint water crisis. It is both a personal account and a clear explanation of how lead contamination happens, how it's detected, and how official denial can delay a response for years.

The Environmental Protection Agency's Safe Drinking Water Hotline and website provide information on lead, PFAS, and other contaminants, including how to find testing resources by state. Available at epa.gov.

The Environmental Working Group's Tap Water Database, also at ewg.org, allows households to look up known contaminants by zip code based on utility-reported data.

On Septic Systems, Sewage, and Rural Infrastructure

The National Environmental Services Center, based at West Virginia University, publishes free, plain-language guides on septic systems, well maintenance, and small community water systems, aimed specifically at homeowners rather than contractors. Available at nesc.wvu.edu.

Underground America: Narratives of the Invisible Infrastructure That Keeps Us Alive, while not a single well-known title, represents a useful category: search for university extension office publications on septic maintenance, which are consistently free, current, and written for general audiences.

On Flooding, Mold, and Housing Health

Toxic Mold Survival Guide by Jeffrey C. May covers mold identification, health effects, and remediation in accessible terms, written by an indoor air quality investigator. It is more practical than alarmist and is directly relevant to the flooding and mold chapter.

The Federal Emergency Management Agency's flood map service at msc.fema.gov allows households to check flood zone status, though as this book notes, flooding can and does happen outside mapped zones.

On Privatization, Utilities, and Public Accountability

Sale of the Century: Russia's Wild Ride from Communism to Capitalism by Chrystia Freeland is not directly about American water, but its account of what happens when public assets are sold off quickly offers useful background for understanding water utility privatization patterns in the United States.

Food and Water Watch, at foodandwaterwatch.org, publishes ongoing research and reporting specifically on water utility privatization, corporate water control, and ratepayer organizing.

On Women, Households, and Environmental Burden

Flint Town on Netflix, also referenced in Book 1, remains directly relevant here as one of the clearest documentary accounts of a water crisis unfolding inside a community, including the household-level labor of managing it.

Erin Brockovich, the film, dramatizes a real groundwater contamination case and remains a useful, accessible entry point for understanding how contamination cases are investigated and fought, even decades later.

Watching

There's Something in the Water on Netflix examines environmental racism and water contamination in Nova Scotia, with themes that translate directly to similar situations across rural and low-income communities in the United States.

PBS Frontline's *Poisoned Water*, available free at pbs.org/frontline, covers the Flint water crisis in documentary detail and pairs well with the contamination chapter.

Listening

Thirst, an investigative podcast series, covers water access, contamination, and infrastructure stories across different American communities, with an emphasis on the people living with the consequences rather than the engineering itself.

99% Invisible, also listed in Book 1, has multiple episodes specifically on water infrastructure, sewer systems, and the history of sanitation, all accessible to general listeners and relevant to several chapters in this book.

Maintenance Phase, also referenced in Book 1, remains useful here for its broader approach to separating systemic failure from personal responsibility, a theme that runs through every chapter of this book.

These resources were current as of the time of writing. Organizations, publications, and streaming availability change. If a specific resource is no longer accessible, a search by title or organization name will usually locate a current version.

About EATMS Productions

What's happening to women now is not random. It's structural.

Policy, culture, technology, and power are moving in the same direction.

EATMS maps them clearly and shows how to respond.

This title is part of an ongoing body of work. All EATMS Productions titles, across all series, authors, and formats, are components of a single connected project.

New titles, series, and resources are added regularly as the project continues to grow.

Start here: EATMS System Primer — Free Bundle https://eatms.gumroad.com/l/dyvzbw

For full catalog or inquiries: eatms.me

Free survival booklet + EATMS updates: email "EATMS" to eatms@pm.me

Please feel free to burn part or all of this book, safely, as an effigy.

www.ingramcontent.com/pod-product-compliance
Lightning Source LLC
Chambersburg PA
CBHW031352230926
51848CB00002B/491
9781966014645